I0478675

What you should know about Cerebral Shunts

The Ventricular System of the Human Brain

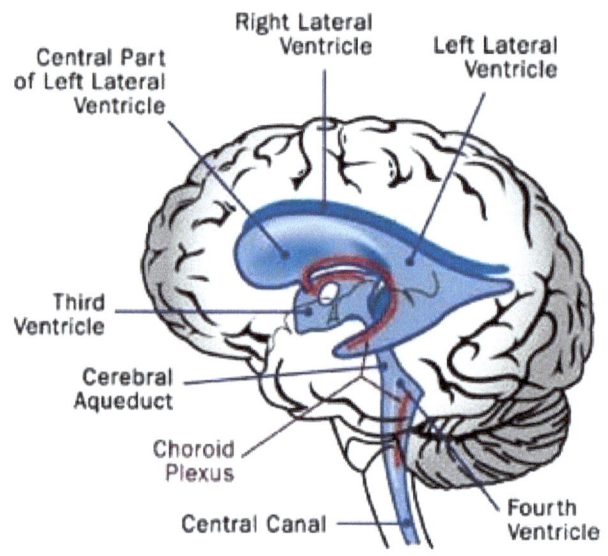

Table of Contents

Dedication's Page

This book is dedicated to all of the medical professionals that help or assist in their patient's recovery.

This book is also dedicated to a friend of mine who will not be named at this time and also to my little cousins and friends who have had the procedure done as well.

Introduction

Hydrocephalus is defined as edema or swelling of a person's brain due to excessive cerebro-spinal fluid(CSF). Cerebral shunts are generally used to treat this type of condition.
If this condition goes unchecked in any way, it may lead to an increase intracranial pressure(ICP).
The increase in intracranial pressure can cause other abnormalities such as herniation, crushed brain tissue and cerebral edema and intracranial hematomas.

Herniation of the Brain

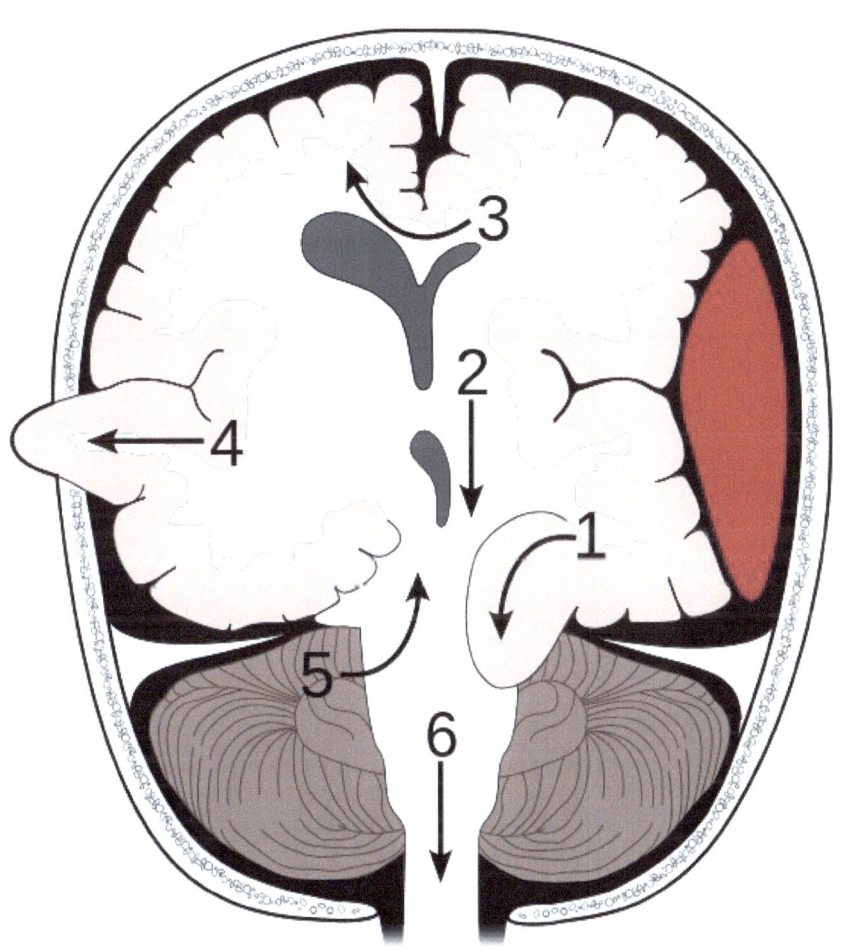

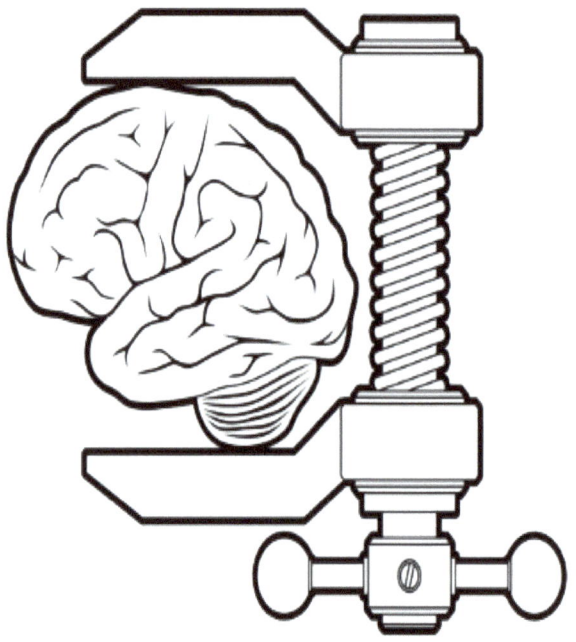

This is what Intracranial Pressure can feel like!!!

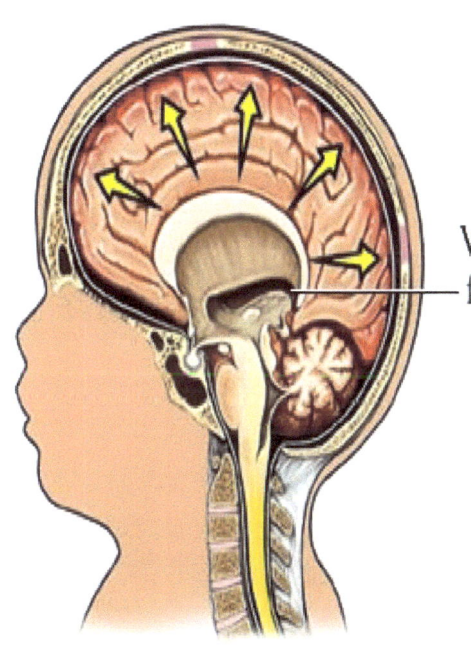

Ventricles fill with
fluid, pushing the
brain outward

A cerebral shunt may be used to prevent or alleviate this or some other similar disease in a patient.

Shunts may come in various forms but generally the shunts have a valve housing that connects to a catheter.

The end of the shunt is placed in the peritoneal cavity.

The Main Differences between Shunts

The main differences between shunts may be as follows:

- Types of valves that may be used in the shunt
- The materials that may be used to construct the shunt
- Whether or not the valve is programmable

Shunt Location

A neurosurgeon usually decides on a shunt's location.

They decide where the blockage is taking place that may be causing the Hydrocephalus.

All of a person's brain ventricles are prime candidates for a shunt's location.

The catheter is usually placed in the peritoneal cavity of the abdomen but a person's heart and lungs may also be used for a shunt's placement.

The Ventricular System of the Human Brain

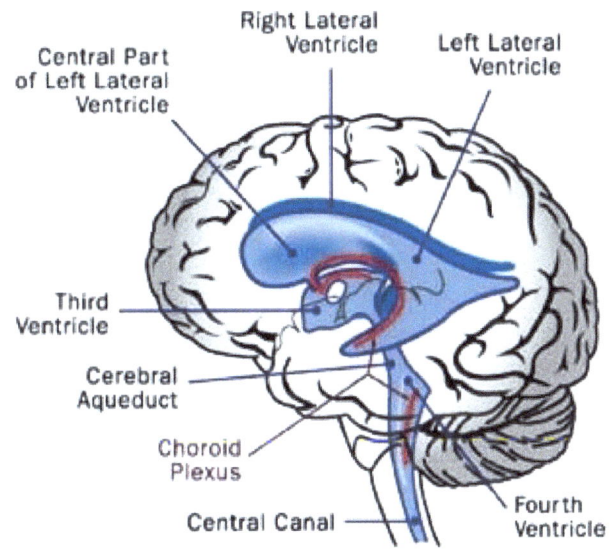

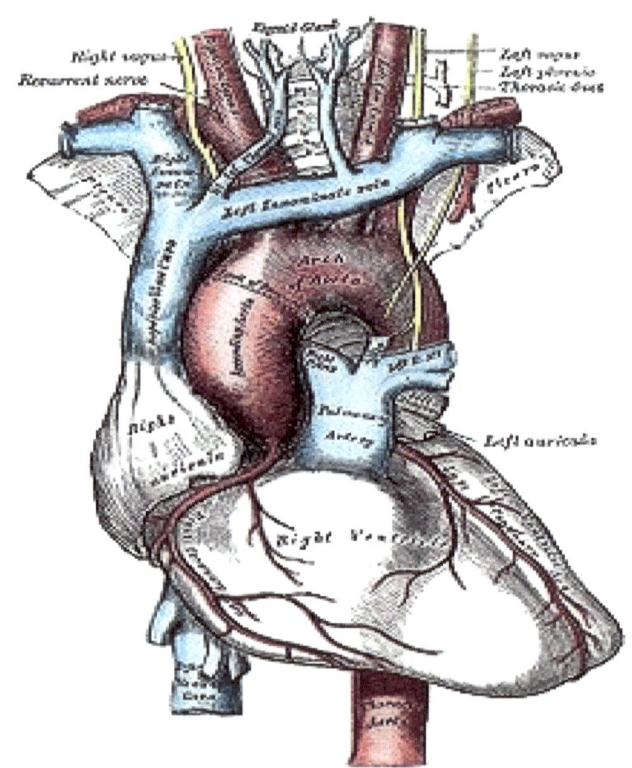

A neurosurgeon may name the route that the shunt has taken.

Any type of tissue can be used as long as they have enough epithelial cells to absorb the incoming (CSF) cerebro-spinal fluid that the tip of the catheter may bring.

Shunt Routing

A ventriculo-peritoneal shunt may be called a VP shunt.

The location of the fluid drain will be the peritoneal cavity.

A ventriculo-atrial shunt may also be called a VA shunt.

The location of the fluid drain may be the right atrium of the heart.

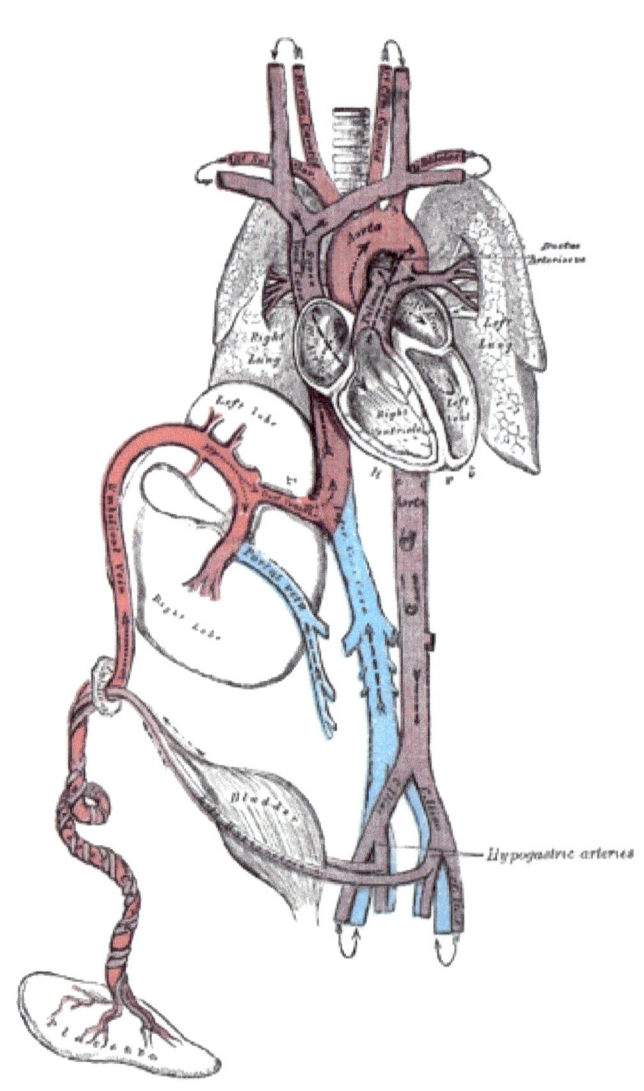

A ventriculo-pleural shunt may be called a VPL shunt.

It is generally placed in the pleural cavity of the human body.

A ventriculo-cisternal shunt could also be called a VC shunt.

This shunt is generally placed in the cisterna magna.

A lumbar-peritoneal shunt may also be referred as a LP shunt.

It is generally placed in the peritoneal cavity as well.

Shunt Complications

Shunt placement may be associated with a number of complications.

Some of these complications generally come during childhood and may dissipate once a person becomes an adult.

Shunt revision(The reprogramming or replacement of an existing shunt) is one of the main complications that a neurosurgeon may come across.

Some common symptoms that may be associated with a shunt revision could be as follows:

- Headaches
- An alternation of consciousness
- Vomiting
- Nausea
- Double-vision

In today's pediatric population, an implantation of a shunt revision two years after the first shunt placement could have a failure rate of 50%.

Infection

Another complication for a shunt placement could be infection.
Generally, this only causes a problem in a pediatric patient due to the patients not having a strong immune system just yet to fight off diseases.
The pediatric patients risk of infection decreases as the patients get older and have built up a stronger immune system over time.

Shunt infection may cause major problems for 27% of the patients that may need a shunt placement.
Shunt infections may lead to other problems such as:
1) Neurological problems
2) Cognitive problems
3) Sometimes, even death

Some common microbial agents used
for Shunt Infections

Common microbial agents that could be
used for Shunt Infections may be:
❖ Candida albicans
❖ Straphylococcus epidermidis
❖ Straphylococcus aureus

Other medical factors that could lead to Shunt Infections

Some other medical factors that may lead to a shunt infection could be having a shunt placement when a patient is very young.
Very young is generally defined as (<6 months of age).
Also, another contributing factor may be the type of Hydrocephalus that may have to be treated.

Other Information

There is no strong correlations between a patient's shunt type and the infection that it may pose on a patient.
Also, a patient could have similar symptoms if they have a shunt infection or Hydrocephalus.
The symptoms could include an elevated white blood count and a high fever.

Some Treatments for a Shunt Infection

Treatments for a CSF shunt infection could include simply removing the shunt until the infection has been resolved and then finding a temporary ventricular reservoir placement until the infection has dissipated.

The Four Main Methods for resolving VP Shunt Infections

There are four main methods for resolving a VP Shunt Infection. The main methods would be:
1) Antibiotic treatments
2) Externalization of the VP shunt with eventual replacement
3) Complete removal of infected shunt with immediate replacement
4) The final method, if done properly, has a 95% successful rate and it is the complete removal of the infected shunt by external ventricular drain (EVD) and eventual shunt re-insertion.

Medical Treatments for Shunt Infections

Some CSF infections may require some initial empiric therapy.

This therapy may include a combination of vancomycin and ceftazidime.

Other additional coverage options could be aztreonam and meropenem because they can be effective for gram-negative bacterial infections.

Surgical Treatments for Shunt Infections

A case study was conducted under Wong, et al in order to produce these statistics. Wong designated two groups for his research. One group would have just medical treatment alone and the other group would have medical and surgical treatment. These groups were observed at the same time.

After the case study was over, Wong suggests that patients be treated by both medical and surgical treatments.

In the past 30 years, 17 case studies have been published about children with CSF shunt infections.

The studies revealed that 88% of 244 infections were resolved by having the shunt removed and then the patient being treated with antibiotics.

However, 33% of 230 shunt infections were resolved by using antibiotic therapy alone.

Another case study that a person could research may be Steinbok, et al.

Obstructions

Obstructions are another leading cause of shunt failures. The blockages are generally found at the proximal or distal ends.
The proximal end of a shunt valve may become obstructed by the build-up of excessive proteins in the CSF fluid.
The extra proteins slowly clog the valve by collecting at the point of the drainage in the shunt.

The distal end of the shunt can also become blocked due to the excessive protein collection or the VP shunt being pulled out of the abdominal cavity.
Some additional causes for blockages or obstructions may be Over Drainage or Slit Ventricle Syndrome.

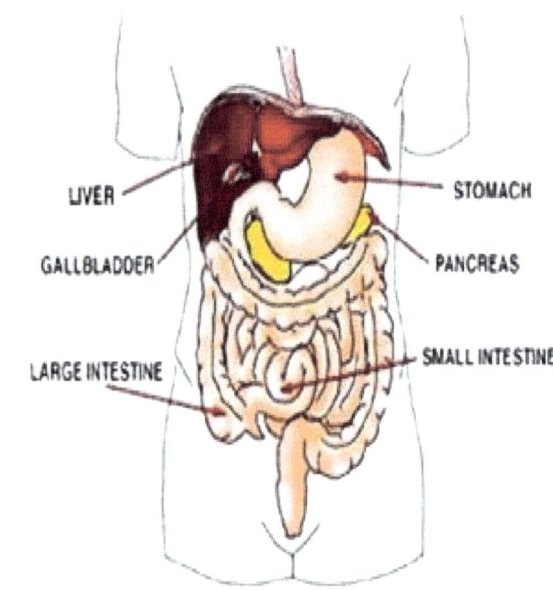

LIVER

STOMACH

GALLBLADDER

PANCREAS

LARGE INTESTINE

SMALL INTESTINE

Over Drainage

Usually, there are two types of over drainage.

The first type is called extra-axial fluid collection.

In this particular condition, a patient's brain may collapse on top of itself caused by blood on the brain or a collection of CSF.

This generally causes severe brain damage by compressing the brain.

A Subdural Hematoma could resort from this condition.

Extra-axial CSF fluid collection may be treated by three methods:

1) The shunt being removed
2) The shunt being reprogrammed
3) The shunt can be reprogrammed so that less CSF is released
4) The fluid will be drained from the brain

Chiari I Malformation

Older studies have thought that Chiari I Malformation was a congenital defect; However, recent studies have shown that Chiari I Malformation is the result of that over drainage of the Cysto-peritoneal shunts that were used to treat Arachnoid cysts could result in overcrowding of the posterior fossa and the development of tonsillar herniation.

Some common symptoms of Chiari I Malformation

The common symptoms of Chiari I
Malformation are as follows:
1) Hearing loss
2) Major Headaches
3) Loss of Cerebellum Function
4) Fatigue
5) Muscle weakness

Slit Ventricle Syndrome

Slit Ventricle Syndrome is often referred to as over drainage and brain growth that occurs simultaneously.

This condition often occurs after a shunt implantation over a period of several years.

With this condition, a patient's brain will fill the intraventricular space thus causing the ventricles to collapse.

The compliance of a patient's brain will decrease and this will not allow the ventricles to enlarge.

This will reduce the patient's chances of curing the syndrome.

By the brain's ventricles collapsing, the shunt valve may become blocked or obstructed in some way.

Slit Ventricle Syndrome is irreversible, therefore, constant care will be necessary for the patient so that they can manage the condition.

The symptoms of this condition are very similar to a shunt's malfunction but there are key differences as well.

The symptoms will appear as cyclical and then they will appear and then the symptoms may subside over a period during a patient's lifetime.

Secondly, the symptoms may be alleviated if the patient lies in a prone position.

Neither postural position nor time will affect the symptoms in the case of a shunt malfunction.

Intraventricular Hemorrhages

During a shunt implantation or revision, an intraventricular hemorrhage can occur at any point and time.
There is a 31% chance of an intraventricular hemorrhage occurring during the surgical procedure for a shunt revision.
This type of condition can cause severe neurological deficiencies as well as a shunt impairment during a shunt implantation or revision.

Conditions that may require a Shunt Placement

Some medical conditions that may require a patient to need a shunt placement may be:

- ➢ Tumors
- ➢ Spina Bifida
- ➢ Congenital Hydrocephalus
- ➢ Dandy-Walker Syndrome
- ➢ Arachnoid Cysts
- ➢ Idiopathic Intracranial Hypertension
- ➢ Craniosynostosis
- ➢ Congenital Aqueductal Stenosis

Conclusions

Although there have been several cases published down through time about patients that may reach "shunt independence", no physician may agree that a patient may ever survive without their shunt placement or shunt revision. Another problem arises with shunt removal because it is very hard to discern when a patient may become shunt independent without very specific conditions. However, shunt removal is rare but it is not an unheard of surgical procedure.

If you or someone you love think that you have any of these symptoms, please consult with your family physician so that they may refer you to a neurologist so that you may consult with them about your symptoms.

The End

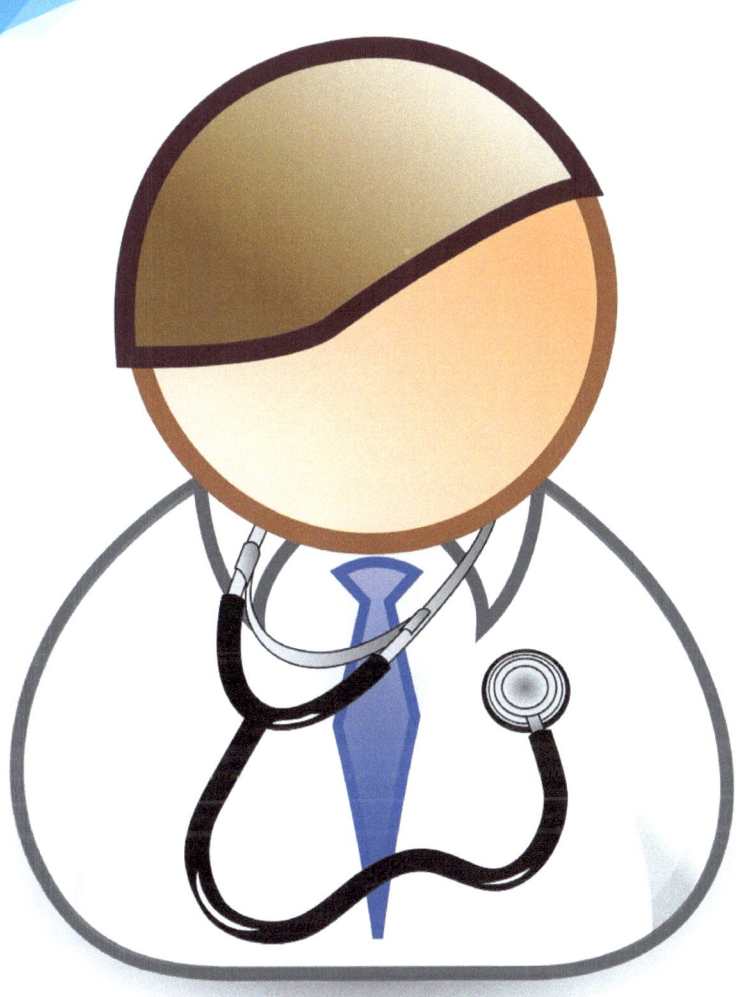

This self-help medical guide gives a person some knowledge that they may need to know about Cerebral Shunts, Their Locations, Symptoms, What they should know about Infection, and Some Diseases that may require a Shunt Placement. If you think that you or someone that you know or love may need one, please consult with your physician as soon as possible.

Misty Lynn Wesley has a very diversified career portfolio in the medical, legal, fashion and insurance industries. She is an avid blogger for Examiner.com, Yahoo Voices, Helium and several others. She also writes articles for CBS Local out of St. Paul, MN and Believe.com on occasion. She is a published author with Publish America and Create Space as well. Her love for her patients and her dual professions were her true inspirations in writing this knowledgeable self-help manual about Cerebral Shunts. God bless!!!

Acknowledgements

The digital art was provided by the following:

1) www.freeillustrations.gatag.net
2) www.lifeinthefastlane.com
3) www.createtohealblogspot.com
4) www.dgcbio.wikispaces.com
5) www.runkle-science.wikispaces.com

Legal Knowledge with the Good Samaritan Law in the United States is necessary before pursuing Arbitration or a Civil Suit.

www.ingramcontent.com/pod-product-compliance
Lightning Source LLC
Chambersburg PA
CBHW050753180526
45159CB00003B/1447